GET YOUR CHILD EATING!

the easy guide to having
Happier Meals
with your kids

Elaine Hodgins

Published in Great Britain in 2017
Under the **HypnoArts** label by
the Academy of Hypnotic Arts Ltd.
1 Emperor Way, Exeter, EX13QS

Hypnoarts.com

Enquiries should be addressed to the
Academy of Hypnotic Arts.
bookpub@hypnoarts.com

First printed edition 2017
British Library Cataloguing in Publication Data
ISBN Number: 978-1-9998921-9-7

Forward

Zoe Clews and Associates Harley Street London

I first met Elaine when I was treating a client for anxiety issues, one of the main reasons for my client's anxiety was her 7 year-old Daughter who point blank refused to eat anything other than chips and mashed potato, getting her to eat anything other than these foods caused intense anxiety and deep distress in the little girl, alarm for her younger sister and exasperation and frustration for her parents.

I hadn't heard of Selective Eating Disorder at the time, my thoughts were that this was a food phobia.

After referring my client's daughter to Elaine, an email 3 months later saying, *"I have no idea how Elaine's done it but my Daughter is now drinking orange juice - even with 'bits in', trying vegetables and her range of foods is growing weekly, the fear has gone and we're all so relieved not to mention amazed!"*.

This issue impacting this entire family, was turned around by Elaine in just a matter of months.

Since recommending that first client to Elaine many years ago I now have the pleasure of knowing Elaine on both a personal and professional level. This book is a natural extension of the warm, caring woman Elaine is.

It is a combination and product of years of experience as a Mother of two, a Paediatric Nurse & Children's Hypnotherapist with an inarguable history of, and stellar reputation for, successfully resolving (SED) Selective Eating Disorder and all its many variations.

Not everyone can get to sessions with Elaine if their child is suffering with SED or picky or fussy eating. Therefore this book is a gift to any struggling parents as it condenses all of Elaine's practical knowledge, tips for parents on how to deal with it & the importance of treating it as quickly as possible.

My client's children refer to Elaine as *'The Magic Lady'* & witnessing their feedback & testimonials, relief & joy at *'getting their children eating'* and the great service for parents she has done here by writing this book, I would be the first to agree. *Magic Lady indeed….*

Zoe Clews

For all the mums, dads and children
I have helped and will continue to help.

For Annie and James who have been,
and always will be... my "raison d'etre"

CONTENTS

Forward by Zoe Clews iii

A NOTE ON HOW THIS BOOK WAS CREATED. 1

INTRODUCTION 3

WHAT IS GET YOUR CHILD EATING?. 5

ELAINE'S STORY 7

WHAT'S GOING ON? 15

   Paediatric Psycho-Therapy PPT And Its Impact
   On Our Emotions 21

   What Causes Emotional Therapy To Get Out
   Of Hand? 27

WHAT CAN WE DO ABOUT IT? 31

WHAT YOU NEED TO DO
   Step 1: Picky or Selective Eating? 35

   Step 2: Understanding Why. 38

   Step 3: If Only It Were That Easy 41

   Step 4: Same Page Positioning 43

   Step 5: TTSBC Planning .46

   Step 6: Glove Puppets And Stories 50

   Step 7: Party Time ... *Not* 58

Step 8: Travel Not Trouble 61

Step 9: Sickness and Safe Foods 65

Step 10: Food Chaining .71

CASE STUDY 1: Alysia Moran 79

CASE STUDY 2: Ethan Crow 89

WHAT ARE THE ALTERNATIVES FOR SED KIDS? 97

MISTAKES, MYTHS AND MISUNDERSTANDINGS
TO AVOID
#1 Myth: No Child Will Starve 103

#1 Mistake: They're Not Naughty 105

#1 Misunderstanding: Behavioural Change Is Easy . .107

MASSIVE MOTIVATION - Have Happier Mealtimes. . . .111

Get Your Child Eating 112

Enjoy A Fuller Future 113

MEET ELAINE. 117

POSTWORD 119

Acknowledgements 121

A note on how this book was created

This book was originally created as a live interview. That's why it reads as a conversation rather than a traditional book that talks "at you". It's also why it isn't after an award for literature but, it will engage, educate and empower you

I wanted you to feel as though I am talking "with you", much like a close friend or relative. I felt that creating the material this way would make it easier for you to grasp the topics and put them to use quickly, rather than wading through hundreds of heavily edited pages.

So relax, and get ready to have Happier Mealtimes with your kids. . .

Elaine

Introduction

Hi everyone and welcome to: Get Your Child Eating covering Emotional Therapy especially for the Mums, Dads and Carer's of children; and, as with all of our experts works, if you want to enhance your experience of life, then there will be advice and techniques you should know and will benefit from…

This is Jonathan Chase for HypnoArts and today I'm talking with Child Psycho-Therapy CPT Expert, Elaine Hodgins, about having happier and less stressful meals with their kids and get the best results.

Elaine has helped hundreds of children with selective eating disorders and other paediatric problems. Working remotely on skype with people as far away as Australia, New Zealand, Canada the USA, Dubai and many places in Europe.

Most of what you need is instruction and encouragement from someone who has "been there and done that!" for an easy guide to having happier meals with your kids.

Elaine Hodgins, thank you for sharing your experience with us on this live interview.

Let's go. . .

What Is Get Your Child Eating?

Elaine: Get Your Child Eating is actually my system of emotional therapy to literally *Get your child eating*.

The book is aimed at being a guide for mums, dads, carers, and obviously children, to help them have a happy family life.

Mealtimes don't need to be nightmares anymore.

Elaine's Story

Jonathan: Okay, Elaine. One thing that everybody likes to understand is how did you get here, helping kids?

Elaine: Right. Well, I came from a background of nursing originally. I did my nursing training many years ago, 1973, and I specialised in paediatrics, so I really got involved with the emotional side of children whilst in hospital, and I really found that quite rewarding.

Seeing a child when they leave hospital and they're well, is *fantastic*.

Then I worked for a time with a Global Airline, and of course seeing children on board the aircraft with food problems, you know, the child is on the plane for 10 hours, hasn't got anything to eat, doesn't like what the airline is offering.

Basically, I got quite used to children being fussy eaters, and that's really how I came into working on emotional therapy with children with eating problems.

Jonathan: How has that progressed into an actual practise?

Elaine: Well, I did my training as a Clinical Hypnotherapist and then opened my first consulting room in Woodley, Berkshire, near to where I live, and the other one in Harley Street in London a couple of years later as I got busier. They've just grown, and I'm seeing probably about 25 children a week now.

Jonathan: I know that you started in generalised practices like other therapists do.

Elaine: Yes, that's right.

Jonathan: What specifically ... I know you're telling me a story. I'm trying to get the specific event that really focused you on kids.

Elaine: Oh, ok. Well, what happened was, I had a lady come to me for weight loss, and we'd done three or four sessions, and obviously, with clients, when they're coming to you for therapy, they do tend to open up to you.

She started to talk to me about her little boy who had a food problem, and wasn't eating very much. He was only eating about six or seven

9

foods. She was quite worried about him, so I said, "Well, you can bring him in. Let's try it." And she brought him in, little Joshua, and yes, he was in quite a bad way. He was only eating six foods, and they were the typical beige, white foods. Bread, pasta, chicken nuggets, that sort of thing. Of course, the poor mother thought that she was to blame.

She felt very guilty, because she thought it was something that she had done wrong. But anyway, I worked with him on the anxiety for food, and of course realised it was a severe food phobia.

With a phobia, obviously what we had to do was reverse the process. I did two or three sessions with him, and after that, he started to eat.

Of course, that mum told other mothers at the school gates, and then I ended up with mostly children coming to see me.

That's really how it all came about.

Jonathan: Now you almost entirely specialise in children.

Elaine: Yes, I would say I see 80% children and 20% adults now at both clinics.

Jonathan: And their families.

Elaine: Yes, and their families. Obviously, I do see ... You know, a child will come to me and then the mum will say, "Could I come to you for weight loss?" Or, "Can my husband come to you for stop smoking?" Of course, I'll see them, because I'm already dealing with the family, but primarily I'm working with children.

Jonathan: Do you work with doctors a lot? Because I know as we share a background in nursing, we don't have that anti-doctor therapeutic problem, do we?

Elaine: No. It's a difficult one, with doctors, because at the moment, especially with the food disorder, it's only just recently been put into the DSMV, which is a Diagnostic and Statistics Manual, that selective eating disorder is actually a condition, a mental condition.

Doctors don't know an awful lot about it as yet. They don't realise that it's a phobia, so of course they're likely to say to the mum or the dad, whoever brings the child to the doctor's, "He's just a fussy eater." And, "Just be more strict with him. Be firmer at the food table, and he'll start eating." Of course, mums are thinking, "I've tried all that. I've done everything he said, but he's still not eating."

They don't really know where to go with it, so I'm working with quite a few doctors at the moment, to educate them in a way, in how phobias with children can be cured, and fairly quickly too!

What's Going On?

Jonathan: What's going on right now in the society that you work in, in the Westernised society, that we're seeing more of this problem of selective eating disorder and picky children?

Elaine: I think, Jon, a lot of the family dynamics have changed over the last 40 to 50 years. I mean, you and I are at an age whereby we sat at the table, didn't we, were given our meal of meat and two veg, and potatoes, and we had to eat our dinner, and we probably didn't get a dessert if we didn't eat it, and that was it.

We all sat down as a family, and that doesn't happen these days so much. I think that's because of the faster pace of life. It's just so much busier. Mums are probably working part-time at least, if not full-time. Children are left with child minders, and that's not a problem.

My own kids went to child minders, and I had to work, because I was a single mum, and I had a child who was a fussy eater.

The problem is, is that things have changed so fast that I don't think the parents can actually keep up with it. They can't understand why their children are being so fussy, picky, about food.

Jonathan: Is that a society thing, do you think?

Elaine: Yes, Well, I think it's environment in general, isn't it? I think it's the environment the child is in.

Naturally, there's so many different family dynamics now, but if you've got your normal family, 2.2 children, and mum's at home, and dad's out working, then you're going to have the mum and dad in the evening having dinner at the table with the family. Everything's fine.

But then if you've got a mum that's a single mum, as indeed I was, who is trying to cope with three children, and two of the children are eating fine, but one of them suddenly starts playing up with food, won't eat, she's going to become very stressed, and she's going to be exhausted trying to cook two or three different meals for the children every day.

Then, I've got one mum, for example, at the moment who I'm seeing at the clinic with her little girl. She's got four children, and she actually cooks four different meals for these children every night, and the poor mum's exhausted herself. If I can help in any way to get those children eating properly, and to ensure that the mum can at least have a calm meal herself at the end of the day, that's really worth something, isn't it?

Jonathan: Can we tell the reader and the listener, watcher, however people are interacting with this interview, can we tell them what *normal eating* means?

Elaine: Is there such a thing?

Normal eating.

Well, normal eating is obviously little Jonny, for example, says he wants some certain breakfast cereal, and mummy says, "No, I haven't got that. You'll have to have Weetabix." Jonny will say, "No, no, no. I don't want it." That's *normal* sort of, "I don't want that. I want ..." Children are like that.

Jonathan: But then he'll eat the Weetabix, because there's no choice.

Elaine: They have likes. They'll still eat the Weetabix, yes, but they have their likes and dislikes just like we do as adults. If they then start getting phobic, obviously, about having to eat something that they've never tried before, then that's a different thing.

If you can see that the child's looking *anxious*, goes *pale*, starts to *gag* if he has to try something that he's never tried before, then you know you're dealing with a child with *selective eating disorder* (SED).

Paediatric Psycho-Therapy PPT And Its Impact On Our Emotions

Jonathan: Elaine, PPT, which is paediatric psychotherapy, what effect does that have on the emotions of your patient, your client?

Elaine: Okay. Well, when a child comes in to see me, they're usually very anxious. Quite scared, really, I suppose, depending on what the problem is.

If it's a food problem, and it's quite a severe one, the child will come in looking very scared, very anxious, and of course the mother's there as well, so her stress and her angst is just overwhelming for the child.

I'm then dealing with a child who's phobic, and also very anxious, and I've also got the mother in the room at the same time, and she's stressed. She could be upset. She could be crying. She's scared.

The therapy is really to help both. It's to help the whole family, in fact, but if the mother and the child are there together, then sometimes I do actually ask the mum to pop out, and I see the child on their own, because they'll tell me more and open up to me.

Obviously, if I'm alone with a child, then I can get them playing with glove puppets and things like that. I make the mum a cup of tea, put her in the waiting room, she sits just outside the room, and I'll chat to the child, and I can get a lot more out of that child this way.

Jonathan: How does it actually affect the emotional process of the child?

Elaine: Right. Well, I think with any therapy, especially when you're dealing with a child's emotions, that's going to be compounded by all the other things going on in the environment.

               For example, the mum being very stressed and worried about the child, that's going to almost say to the child's subconscious mind, "Well, there's a problem here. I've got a disorder. I must be quite seriously poorly." You know?

               The therapy, I think, helps to calm that down. It helps to focus the child's mind on perhaps looking at ways to get that child eating.

               Looking at it like a little project for the child, you know? Giving them a reward chart, and saying, "Look, chart down how many foods you're eating, how many you want to eat." I think the therapy just focuses that child's mind, and really helps the emotions, and calms the situation down.

Of course, most mums have already tried reward charts but when the child is now accountable to me and not the mum it's a whole different ball game.

Jonathan: What is that emotional process that you're looking to achieve?

Elaine: I guess in a way, we're just reversing the process. The best way I can explain it is, imagine you're the child. You be the child, okay? I would say to you, "Jonathan, in your head, imagine that you've got living there two little dinosaurs. Two little minuscule dinosaurs.

One is called *Naughtyosaurus*, and one is called *Smartosaurus*.

Now, the *Naughtysaurus* is the one that says to you, "We don't want to eat that. That food looks disgusting! It looks horrible."

But the *Smartosaurus* is the clever one, and he's the one that's going to be saying to you, "Actually, you haven't even tasted it yet. Why don't you just taste it?"

These two are always at loggerheads. They're fighting with each other, and so it's my job really, now, to help you to sort these two out.

Basically, we've got to kick that *Naughtysaurus's* butt right out of there and get him out. That's really how I work with children. It's how I explain it to the child and the mum.

Jonathan: Right. You're using visualisation
                  techniques and that sort of thing.

Elaine: Yes, that's right Jon.

What Causes Emotional Therapy To Get Out Of Hand?

Jonathan: I know this is hard to explain technically, but as a parent, I'm concerned about what effect does that have on my child's emotional states?

Elaine: Right.

Jonathan: What does that actually do in their head?

Elaine: Okay. Well, it's not going to do any harm. Let's put it that way. All I'm doing is trying to alleviate the anxiety, to be honest with you. It's trying to get rid of their anxiety, because once we've got rid of the fear then they're more likely to try food, new foods.

Once they start trying the foods, and they realise the foods aren't going to hurt them, they're actually going to be okay.

I work with children with all sorts of different phobias. It's no different really, from working with somebody who's got a spider phobia, or a fear of flying.

Phobias all really work on the same sort of premise of trying to reverse that process, get rid of the fear, get rid of the panic.

Quite often, people go into a panic attack. If they've got a phobia, they'll go into a panic attack, and it actually starts that whole sort of vicious circle of panic, have the phobia, panic again, then you panic that you're going to have a panic attack. It's just never ending.

We've got to get them out of the

loop, basically. We've got to stop that loop keep going around.

Jonathan: Then once they've been through the process, they are averagely normal?

Elaine: Very normal, I would think, yep. But I mean, a child is a child.

They're going to have foods that they don't like, just like you and I have got foods we don't like. I don't like most vegetables, but I wouldn't admit that to anybody, so don't tell anybody. (LOL) At the end of the day, some children like some foods, and some like others.

You've got to get back to that normal sort of average.

Jonathan: It's not an abnormal change in their emotions.

Elaine: No, not at all.

What Can We Do About It?

Jonathan: Okay. Right. Elaine, the parents sitting at home reading this, looking at it, and now they are asking: "What do I do now?"

Elaine: Okay. Well, the first thing is, is **not** to panic. **Stop** feeling guilty, because that's what most mums do when their child doesn't eat.

It's a mother's nature to nurture her child, so when the child doesn't eat, she gets very upset, she gets very anxious, and if you're in a state, you're not going to be able to help your child. If you're anxious, and you're stressed, and you're exhausted, you're not going to be in the best place mentally to get your child eating, so the best thing you can do right now is *sit down*, have a *cup of tea*, and make yourself a little *plan* of what you're going to do.

Perhaps the next meal comes along, you could just *observe* your child. See how many foods he's eating, see how he reacts when you give him a new food, but don't make a big fuss about it. Just let it go, and then just play it by ear over the next few days.

Make some notes, because if you go to see a professional like me, they'll ask you questions, and they'll need to know the answers.

They'll need to know *how long* your child has been like this, *how many foods your child is eating,* and *how much he weighs.*

Does he get anxious about other things in his life? Because usually there's two or three things that perhaps are associated. Has there been any change in his life recently? Has there been a *new sibling arrived,* or *house move,* or you've been away on holiday, or has a *pet died* or something? Could be something like that, and it might be just a short-lived thing, which we could perhaps get through quite quickly.

However, if it goes on and continues, then naturally the child will need professional help.

Jonathan: You're saying don't make mealtimes a battle.

Elaine: I'm saying don't make mealtimes a

battle at the moment, because there will come a time where you'll have to be a bit more assertive, but I would rather you be a bit more assertive when you're not so anxious and upset, because otherwise it will turn into a battle again.

Jonathan: And to observe.

Elaine: And to observe, yes.

What You Need To Do

Step 1: Picky or Selective Eating?

Jonathan: Okay, Elaine. Now we've got some steps and stages that the parent can follow. What's stage one, step one?

Elaine: Okay. **Step one** would be for you to find out if your child's just a picky eater, or a selective eater, i.e. has your child got SED - selective eating disorder. To do that, I'd ask you five questions.

First one would be, does he or she eat less than 10 foods?

The second one would be, does he gag when trying a food, or gag, or retch? I don't know what people describe that as.

The third one would be, did your child ever suffer reflux as a baby? Because that quite often happens.

The fourth one is your child brand-specific or colour-specific when it comes to food?

The last one would be, does he appear anxious when he's eating? That's actually probably the most important one. *Is your child anxious when he is trying a new food?*

With those questions, if you get the answer "yes" to all of them, obviously he's eating less than 10 foods, "yes," he's more likely to have selective eating disorder, and not be just picky.

A child with picky eating can be bribed. He can be cajoled. He can be encouraged to eat.

You could say to that child, "I'll buy you a great big box of Lego if you eat this piece of broccoli," and yes, he'll eat it. That's the picky eater. He'll eat it, because he wants the Lego.

But if you offered the child who's got a selective eating disorder, if you offered him a holiday in Disney World, Disney Land, he wouldn't. *He still wouldn't eat.* He would rather starve. That's the difference between the picky and the selective.

Step 2: Understanding Why

Jonathan: Fabulous. Now, step two.

Elaine: Okay. **Step two** is all about understanding your child as a picky eater. Now, what could happen is that certain things could happen at home, like a new baby may have arrived, or something going on. The house is being renovated, lots of workmen around, all sorts of things.

He could be just copying an older sibling, an older sibling who's pretending to be fussy at the table. He could be just wanting to be clever like the big brother, as boys do, or girls, and he could have been hospitalised, and then been in hospital, come out of hospital, doesn't want to eat. Probably a bit anxious.

You've got all these things going on, so if you've had a lot of angst going on with the child, then you can sit down and say, "Ah, it's probably because of that. Well, okay. Let's sort that out then."

If it's because a new baby has arrived, let's give him a little bit more attention. Or if it's because the older boy, the older brother is playing up or something, let's have a talk to him, and let's calm that situation down.

You can probably sort these little things out yourselves just by having a chat with the child, with the siblings. Having a family chat, really.

Of course, there will be a certain amount of control that comes into the child's eating, because as the child develops, he's learning independence. He wants to assert his control. That's up to you to be a little bit assertive with him, and say, *"Okay, well you say you don't like it, but you haven't tried it yet. Let's try it first and see."*

But again, you can only do this if you're not anxious yourself.

Step 3: If Only It Were That Easy

Jonathan: Okay. I resonate with the title of the next step.

Elaine: Okay. ***If only it were that easy.***

Yes. That's what every mum says to me.

When they come to me at the clinic, when I'm talking to them about the child, and ask them if they've tried certain things, and suggest little things to do, they say, "If only it were that easy."

Of course, it is difficult. No parent wants to see their child anxious.

No child wants to get anxious themselves around the mealtime, because mealtimes should be a time when the family are together, and having a nice hour at least to have a chat about their day, and it's good for the children psychologically to do that.

But now that you've established how serious your child's eating is, whether it's picky eating or whether he's actually got an eating disorder, now there's certain things that we can do to ... We can start a plan.

Let's make a plan. That's the first thing.

Step 4: Same Page Positioning

Jonathan: Right. Step four.

Elaine: **Step four is Same Page Positioning.** Basically, we need to be working on the same page.

Let's make a plan.

First, talk to other siblings, brothers and sisters who might be ridiculing your child. They might be saying, "You're a picky eater. You don't eat this. You don't eat that." It's going to upset the child, so get them on side. Get everybody on side.

Have a main meal together at least two or three times a week. Perhaps it's not possible to do it every night.

I know it's difficult with mum's and

dad's both working, but at least two or three times a week, have a meal together. … in that way your child can then see food on the table.

He can see what other people are eating, he can hear others talking about food and how yummy it is… and if you have to, arrange a meeting with the teacher so that the lunchtime problem can be sorted out, so the child, if he's been picky at school, will know that the teacher or the dinner lady knows that he perhaps can't eat certain foods, maybe you could explain to the teacher that he's a little bit picky and he might need a little bit more encouragement to eat.

Really make mealtimes light hearted, you know? Make them fun. Have a chat, and just be calm.

Get rid of all that angst at the table, the tension, the stress that's been happening obviously over a period of time. I think that's what same page positioning is. It's working all together as a team, everybody reading off the same page.

Step 5: TTSBC Planning

Jonathan: Number five.

Elaine: **Step five, TTSBC Planning.**

"What's that?" I can hear you ask.

Well, it stands for *Taste*, *Texture*,
Smell, *Brand* and *Colour*. All these
things are what we look at in a
child with an eating disorder.

Now, we need to establish what it
is that your child gets upset about
with food, so for example, it could
be just the taste, or it could be just
the texture. Some children have
sensory processing disorder, which
is all about the senses. It could be
that he has an extra sensitive smell,
and so certain foods just make him
feel awful when he smells them –
fish for example, or eggs!

Brand, we've already discussed a little bit on brand, but when a child is told about certain brands of food every day on the television, obviously it's sticking in his mind just as the manufacturer wants it to! He's going to remember that brand, and perhaps ask for it all the time, and if mum gives it to him all the time, what's going to happen?

And *colour*. That is a big one.

Most of the children who are eating very few foods, you'll find that they're eating white, beige foods. Carbohydrates, pasta, rice, bread. This means that of course the child won't lose weight. Even though he's not eating that well, so that when you do take him to the doctor's, he's actually not lost any weight, which is quite interesting, isn't it? Because we're thinking that our children are not eating well, but they're not losing weight.

When you do take them to the doctor and they haven't lost any weight, the doctor will say, "*Well, he's fine. He hasn't lost any weight.*"

What I would do next is to make a list of your child's safe foods.

If there are only six, seven safe foods, then look at them and see what they are. Are they *savoury*? Are they *sweet*? Are they *crunchy*? Are they *dry*? Are they *wet* foods?

Try and establish what type of foods your child is eating at the moment, and what they have eaten in the past.

Jonathan: What do you mean specifically by "safe"?

Elaine: Ah, safe foods. Yes – sorry Jon.

            This is what the child tends to call
            their foods. They're their safe
            foods that they eat, that they like,
            and mum tends to call them a safe
            food, because she knows that if
            they go anywhere, and they have
            that child's particular safe food,
            then it's safe for the child.

            It's just a term that mums use.

Step 6: Glove Puppets And Stories

Jonathan: Number six.

Elaine: **Number six. Glove Puppets and Stories.**

Yes, well having worked with children almost all my life anyway, and having two kids of my own, and two grandchildren, I use glove puppets a lot.

Glove puppets and stories, games, anything to really distract the child to have fun, to have a good time, and whilst I'm doing that, whilst I'm talking with the glove puppets, and I've usually got one on the child and one on me, so we're having a conversation, that child is talking to ... He's talking to the glove puppet, he's talking to *Mickey*

Meerkat, or *Marvin Monkey*. He's not really talking to me, so he's more likely to be more open and tell me things that he probably wouldn't normally tell me, like why he doesn't want to eat that certain food.

If you had a couple of glove puppets, and you played with your child with the glove puppets, just having normal little games, normal little conversations, even telling them a story about some animals who had some eating problems, a monkey that didn't like eating bananas, for example, or a donkey that didn't like eating carrots, something like that.

Talk to your children, have fun with them, play with them.

There's lots of games that you can buy that are related to food items;

Shopping List, Pop to the shops, etc. or games to do with food that you can play with them. You could even buy some plastic fruit, vegetables.

There's lots of different things that you can do as a mum to help your child, using glove puppets, stories, games and role play – even singing songs about food.

Here is a little story:

Ella's Magic Flowers. (suitable for children from 2-7 years old)

Ella went out in the garden. She liked the garden because it was full of pretty colourful flowers. She would talk to the flowers and they would talk back to her. She called it her Magic Garden because it had Magic Flowers that used to talk to her and help her with her problems.

"Hello Ella" said the Red Flower. "How are **you** today?"

"Well" she said, looking a bit sad, "I'm not feeling very happy today".

"Oh dear why not?" asked the pretty Red Flower.

"Because I'm a bit worried about trying new food "she sighed.

"Well" said the Red Flower "We had better get you **nice and calm, so you *don't* worry about that hadn't we!**"

"Mmmmm…."

"The problem is, I keep thinking I'm not going to like it" she said.

"Well, we can soon put that right. Touch my petals! Then, when you hear a "**PING**" you will know you have the super magic power to be confident and taste the food!" said the red magic flower! (*Mum – say Ping when the child touches the petals!*)

Ella gently touched the Magic Red Flower's petals.

PING!

There was a little sound coming from the flower and it lit up very brightly!

"Thank you" said Ella, smiling, and she walked on further down the garden.

"Hello Ella!"

She looked down and saw a pretty blue flower.

"Hello" she said

The Blue Flower looked up at her. She said: "I heard you talking to Red Flower about your worry about tasting food and I thought I may be able to help too! I am a magic Blue Flower and if you touch my petals I will give you the power to have loads of **self-belief** so that you will just *know* you can do it!"

She touched Blue Flower's petals.

PING! The magic flower had given Ella her special power!

"Thank you, Blue Flower – you are *very* kind!"

Ella walked down to the bottom of the garden thinking about it all and how wonderful it was going to be when she tasted all the new food.

"Hello Ella" It was the Magic Yellow Flower! "I heard what the red flower and the Blue flower said. I can help you too. If you touch my magic petals, they will give you the power to **do whatever you want to do.**"

"That's really kind of you Yellow Flower. I would really like to be able to do that" said Ella

"In that case you *know* what to do!" said the flower.

She touched the pretty petals and...

PING! The magic was done!

"Thank you flowers! Thank you to **all** the flowers in my Magic Garden!"

She ran back to the house with a huge **smile on her face**. Her mummy said: "Hello Darling where have you been?"

"I've been to my Magic garden Mummy. My friends, the Magic Flowers are all going to help me to try new foods".

Mummy smiled. "Wow! That's **fantastic!**"

Mummy prepared the tea! Ella sat at the table.

she tasted a new food - "Mmmmm" she said, "It's ok"

Then she had her bath and cleaned her teeth and got ready for bed. She had a lovely story and then mummy tucked her down, tucking her duvet around her nice and cosy! She closed her eyes.................. and she dreamt she was in a restaurant choosing lots of different foods! And the three magic flowers in the garden all winked at each other...and went to sleep! Their job was complete! Goodnight!

All mum has to do is buy some artificial flowers, three different colours, to use as props for the story.

When it gets to the part about the magic powers – get your child to touch the flowers – thereby giving him/her a super power to make her less anxious so he/she will eat.

It *does* work! Keep the flowers in the kitchen or dining room so they are always handy at mealtimes!

If you are creative you can make up similar stories utilizing the things that your child likes!

Step 7: Party Time ... Not

Jonathan: Elaine, moving on, number seven.

Elaine: Okay. **Step seven is "Party time ... NOT!."**

Children love birthday parties, don't they? But *not* the child who has selective eating disorder.

We've been talking about a child being picky, a child being a little bit fussy, but this is a whole different ballgame.

This is a child who will get totally anxious if he's thinking about going to his best friend's birthday party. He desperately wants to go, desperately, but he can't, because there might not be the food there that he likes.

He might not have a safe food. The other children might make comments.

Party time for children with selective eating disorder is not very happy. You see, he would be anxious, overwhelmed. He would be in such a state, and that's if ... only, if mum can get him there in the first place – most little children with selective eating disorder will just refuse point- blank to go!

Mentally and emotionally, it's not good for your child, because we don't want him or her to miss out on socialising with other children. That's how they learn.

The older child with SED, they can almost become agoraphobic. They will refuse to go to a party, refuse to go out to dinner, refuse to go out to lunch with mum and dad and some friends, because they know that there's going to be tension at the table.

The older child can even get depressed, and perhaps just stay in their room. Some of them even resort to self- harming. It's very difficult for children to socialise.

When I say: "*party time*," I'm not literally meaning a birthday party, but I'm trying to get across that it's not fun for children.

Step 8: Travel Not Trouble

Elaine: Okay. **Step eight. Travel, Not Trouble.**

Now, with a child with selective eating disorder, I do insist, I do say that you should get help, because it can be quite serious, and going from being a picky eater to having selective eating disorder is a very big stage.

We're going to talk about going on holiday with a child with SED.

It would probably be your biggest nightmare, but that's if you actually got it to happen at all. Because when you go away with a child, and you go on holiday, you've got to remember so many things.

You've got to remember: ***Will there be the food on the aircraft, to start with, that the child would actually eat? What if I can't buy my child's safe food abroad?***

Most mums worry that if their child stops eating whilst on holiday – he just won't start again when they get home!

It can move quite fast from a child eating just two or three foods, to eating **nothing**.

Do I need to take a suitcase full of chicken nuggets or something? If I do take food with me, is it allowed in? Because if you're going to somewhere like Australia or some places in America, there's certain foods you can't take in anyway.

There's quite a lot to think about when you're travelling with a child anyway, but with a child who hardly eats anything and is specific about what he *does* eat – its ten times harder!

I know some mums say to me, "Do you know what? It's not even worth us going on holiday. It's too much trouble, because whenever we go away, we're all anxious. It's just an absolute nightmare."

Those are their words. What will happen if you do take your child away and there's no food? That's a mother's big dilemma. There's no food for your child to eat. What is that child going to eat? Yes, they'll find him some bread, a few chips maybe, and okay, it probably won't hurt him for a week, but if you're away for two or three weeks, that child's going to be pretty anxious and hungry!

You know, he's not going to be very healthy at the end of that holiday. It's worth thinking about where you go for your holiday when you've got a child who's got selective eating disorder. But better still, get the selective eating disorder sorted out – *fast!*

Step 9: Sickness and Safe Foods

Jonathan: Number nine.

Elaine: **Step nine: Sickness and Safe Food.**

Probably sickness in a child with selective eating disorder is every parent's dread.

What do we do when a child who's not taking very much anyway stops eating because he's poorly? It's a real dilemma for you as a mum.

If they can drink milk, brilliant. Any milk he drinks. Hot chocolate, cold chocolate. It doesn't matter, as long as they're drinking some sort of fluid. Lots of water.

When it comes to medicines, and

this is a bit of a grey area with some mums, because I've had mums call me and say, "My child needs medicine, but she won't take it."

Now, I have one rule, and I had it with my children as well, is that food is one thing, medicine is another.

I would say to you as a mum, if your child had meningitis and he had to take some medicine for him to survive, what would you do? They always say, "I'd get the medicine down. I'd make sure she took that medicine."

Well, this is exactly the same. If a child is sick and he needs medicine, then he should take that medicine, and you've got to do whatever you need to do to get that medicine down, and push fluids, because normally when a child is poorly, they get dehydrated and they need fluids – ***lots of them!***

I'll tell you a little story from my past, when I was a nurse a long time ago. I was working in the A and E dept., and it was Christmas Eve, a mum came running in with a child in her arms. She was about 18 months old, little blond curls, gorgeous little thing, but I could see she was critical.

I grabbed her, took her into the crash room, resus room, and pressed the crash bell.

The team came, and they worked to save that child for probably well over an hour, but sadly they failed.

They couldn't save the little girl.

I'd taken the mum into the family room, given her a sweet cup of tea, as we did in those days - I think we still do now - and had a chat with her, and she'd explained to me that the child, for a few days, had had a tummy bug or gastroenteritis, some form of diarrhoea and vomiting.

I said, "Did you take her to the doctor's?"

"Yes. Got a prescription for some medicine."

"And you gave her the medicine?"

"Well, she wouldn't take it. She's very picky. She wouldn't take the medicine."

"And what about fluids? Did you give her any water or anything?"

"Well, no. She didn't want it, so I didn't push it."

That little girl died basically of dehydration, simply because the mum wouldn't push those fluids, and didn't want to give her the medicine because the child said she didn't want it!.

I get very, *very* ... What's the word? *Stern*! with mums about this, because I think food is one thing, drinks are another thing, but actually medicine is very, *very* important.

If the child has to take medicine, he or she **has got to have it**, no matter how you get that medicine down them.

There's lots of different ways now anyway, with suppositories, and at the worst, they have to have an injection. The fear of having an injection alone will probably make them have the medicine.

That's when we're talking about sickness and safe foods, *this* is what I mean.

If the child is only having five or six safe foods, and they suddenly get sick, they suddenly get ill, they might not want to eat.

There's that fear that they might not go back to those six foods, and they might stop eating, so you've got to be really careful about just keeping their diet bland, keep encouraging them to eat the things they already are eating.

Don't bother about pushing them with new foods at this stage. *Wait until they're better.*

Step 10: Food Chaining

Jonathan: Okay. Fabulous. Thank you.
Moving on, the next thing we can
do.

Elaine: Okay. **Step 10 would be food
chaining.**

Now, food chaining is just exactly
as it says. It's *chaining* or *linking* one
food to another.

What we want to do is to link the
foods that your child's already
eating, or the foods that he *used* to
eat and has since stopped, to new
foods.

For example, if he's eating chicken
nuggets, which is a bit of chicken
and breadcrumbs, he obviously
likes the crunchy breadcrumbs.

71

Why not try him with fish fingers in breadcrumbs? And if he's eating yogurt, which is obviously a smooth, wet consistency, why not try him with custard? It's basically linking foods that he's already eating to new foods. That's the simplicity of it.

A lot of mums don't think about it in that way. They just say, "Oh, what can I give my child to eat?"

What I would suggest to you as a mum is to make a list of the foods that your child likes, and whether that's six foods or 60, it doesn't really matter. Just make a list of them, and put down the foods that he used to eat, because a lot of children will drop foods, and then they pick them back up again at a later date.

Then *find* foods, just sit and think of foods that are very similar, and talk to your child, let him help you.

Let's say, "Come on, tell me, what do you think is similar to this that you might like?" Involve your child.

Make it a *game* — make it *fun*!

That's what he needs. Take him to the supermarkets. Let him choose what *he* wants to eat. We all like to choose what we want to eat, don't we really? Take him to the supermarket.

Get cooking with them. Do lots of food stuff with them. Food play, all that sort of thing.

Once the child is around food a lot more, sees food on the table a lot more, plays with food, talks about food, it'll be hard not to eat it, won't it? That's food chaining.

Jonathan: How will you know when you've got results.

Elaine: Okay. By now, you will have established whether your child is a picky eater or a child who is suffering with selective eating disorder.

Whichever it is, this book is obviously going to help you get your child eating.

How will you know when you've got results?

Well, the first thing will be that your child won't be anxious. He won't be anxious around food, sitting at the table, chatting about food. Sometimes when you talk to a child even about food, they clam up and they go anxious. But if you're getting results, then your child won't be anxious about food.

I had a lady just recently call me.

We were talking about something else, and I said, "Oh, how's little Sebby getting on? How's his food progress coming along?"
And she said, "Well, you know what? He hasn't tried that many new foods, but I can see such a huge difference in him.

He's not anxious around food. Instead of having thrown a complete tantrum if I ask him to try something, he'll just say, "No, not at the moment, mummy."
Which is totally different to what he used to do, so I can see that as a big sort of improvement."

That's the type of results that you'll
start to see. You might see that
first, before the child even starts
eating food.

The child might feel happier when
you're going out to eat, say for
example if you go out for lunch,
you go to a restaurant.

Sometimes the child will play up.
Children play up anyway in
restaurants, don't they? But the
child will play up because there's
nothing for him to eat. None of his
safe foods are there, but he might
just sit down and start trying food,
and you'll probably be so shocked
you'll need a glass of wine to get
over it, but that's what they do,
and they surprise you.

When they pick up a food with no
problem at all, and just start eating

it, that's when you know you've got real results.

Here's a case study of one of my little kiddies – I have permission from her and mum to use their names.

Case Study 1:
Alysia Moran

History:

Session 1: Alysia came to see me with her mum - Anita Reed. A lovely, polite little girl who looked very thin and pale, and extremely anxious.

Anita (mum) explained to me that Alysia had been a picky eater since being a toddler but that the situation had gradually become worse over the past year and she was now only eating (or rather drinking) chocolate milkshake and strawberry drinking yogurt. No solid food at all as she was so scared of choking!

She was losing weight and mum was extremely worried. The doctors had appeared not to be too worried but Anita knew that this was getting more severe so she had decided to bring her to see me.

Alysia has two older siblings and comes from a very loving family. She was doing well at school, was very outgoing, had lots of friends and was a very fun-loving girl, but mum had noticed she was becoming more withdrawn. They couldn't go out to eat as a family as there would be nothing Alysia could eat and it caused tension whilst they were out. Mum had had to talk to the teachers at her school because they had become aware of Alysia's struggle with food.

I used some games and role play to build rapport with her and then we talked about her fear of food.

The only thing she could really explain to me was that she was scared she was going to choke every time she ate something. I used a few little hypnotic techniques with her to work on her subconscious mind so that the fear and anxiety of food would start to subside. I also gave her a reward chart to fill in. (children love these!) explaining to her that I wanted her to try three foods a week and when she tried one she would get a sticker. So many stickers would get her a little treat.

Session 2:

Alysia and her mum came in and mum explained that there hadn't been much change.

Alysia was still very scared to eat but she had at least tried a few foods i.e. putting them in her mouth and chewing them but couldn't bring herself to swallow them.

We talked about school and her home life in general and everything seemed fine. She wasn't being bullied at school, home life was lovely and she didn't appear to be worried about anything. She was sleeping very well but had a few problems with constipation due to the lack of fibrous food and possibly not enough liquids.

We did some parts therapy, asking that pesky little *Naughtysaurus* in her head who was telling her not to eat, to leave her alone and allow the *Cleversaurus* to give her good advice about food! She told me that "*she had asked the Cleversaurus to kick the butt of the Naughtysaurus right outta her head – but he kept coming back*"

She had also filled in the reward chart – she had been able to put the foods into her mouth and chew them but still couldn't bring herself to swallow them.

I sent her a couple of little recordings that she could listen to that would relax her and the metaphorical stories would perhaps touch something in her subconscious mind to allay her fear about the food.

I suggested to mum for the next session I would see Alysia on her own. (Mum was just waiting outside the door in my waiting room with a cup of tea). This would perhaps allow her to open up to me a little more.

Session 3:

Alysia and her mum came in and she seemed quite anxious as she knew we may be trying some food at this session.

Mum popped out and we did some work with metaphorical stories and had a little chat about how **well** she was doing with putting the food in her mouth and we were only one step away now from swallowing the food!

She tried a small piece of tuna sandwich but gagged and had to spit it out so we then tried the chocolate soft cookie. She gagged a little at first but with some encouragement she ate a small piece.

This was a huge step.

She now knew she could swallow something without choking. I told Anita to concentrate on food chaining (linking foods that Alysia used to eat that she could now try again)

Session 4:
Mum reported that Alysia had been trying many more foods and was now eating sausage rolls, cookies, yogurt, tuna sandwiches and a couple of other things that she used to eat.

This was a fantastic result. She had put on some weight and was starting to look a lot healthier.

As my programme is normally 4 sessions taken fortnightly – we decided to give her a break from the sessions for a good month.

However, I explained to Anita and Alysia that she still had to try at least three new foods a week. There would be some that perhaps she wouldn't like but there would almost certainly be some that she *would* like.

It's a numbers game and even if she only liked one new food a week – over a year that's 52 new foods added to her diet!

Session 5: (one month later)
I hardly recognised Alysia when she bounced into my clinic that day. She looked healthier.

She had certainly put on weight and she was full of beans – very chatty and smiley and telling me all about school and her friends!

A very different girl to the pale, thin, sad, little one that had walked into my room that day!

She was eating normally – she was happy – mum was delighted and the rest of the family were happy too!

They had been out to restaurants for meals and Alysia could now eat something off the menu.

They also went on a family holiday and had '*the best time in many years*' because food was no longer a problem.

Alysia's food phobia and general anxiety had completely gone.

What Alysia's Mum says:

"Hi, my name is Anita Reed and when I made the appointment to see Elaine, my daughter Alysia was eating just two foods – well – drinking really – *not* eating! Strawberry drinking yogurt and chocolate milkshake.

She had difficulty swallowing those and she even had difficulty swallowing her own saliva. She used to hold the saliva in her mouth and keep a tissue in her hand and spit it out every now and then as she was so scared to try and swallow.

On the first session, Elaine put myself and Alysia at ease straightaway and seemed to understand Alysia within the first ten minutes of meeting her – she just *got it*.

On the second session, Elaine managed to get Alysia eating a small piece of chocolate chip cookie. This sounds a very small thing but it was a *huge* step for Alysia! Then a small tuna sandwich ....and it just continued after that!

Elaine worked exceptionally hard with both me and Alysia and always made me feel more confident in dealing with my daughters Selective eating disorder. I always left her clinic feeling so much calmer and at ease.

I think Elaine managed to get Alysia eating by giving her little techniques on how to deal with her food anxiety and her fears of swallowing.

She really made Alysia feel so much more confident so that she believed that she *could* eat. Elaine always listened to Alysia and was always very patient and reassuring with her.

She always stayed in touch, in between the sessions and even after the programme had ended, supporting both of us as I needed her help too!

Before we saw Elaine, Alysia had lost all her confidence. She was a sad little girl and didn't go and play with her friends. The rest of the family and our friends didn't recognise her.

She had gone into her shell and we just couldn't do anything to help her. I felt so useless. I felt I had completely lost my little girl. Now, since her sessions with Elaine she is a different child! She's confident, fun loving, happy and everyone has noticed the change. She has also put on weight and looks so healthy.

We, (the whole family) can't thank Elaine enough for what she has done for our family. Alysia is well and happy again and I have my lovely little girl back.

Anita Reed, (Alysia's Mum)

Case Study 2:
Ethan Crow

Session1:

Ethan came to see me with his mummy Michelle because he had been slowly reducing the foods that he had once liked, and Michelle was worried that the situation was getting worse.

Ethan hadn't always been a fussy eater but after a choking incident at two years old he had gradually stopped eating all his favourite foods!

Now, as he was getting older he was now refusing even to try new foods or even the foods that he used to eat.

He was the youngest child in the family, two older sisters, mum and dad, so mum knew the difference from having two daughters that had good appetites to having a little one who was scared to eat.

Ethan was very quiet during that first session. He sat at my little kiddie's table and did some colouring whilst I chatted to him. I didn't mention too much about food on that first session as I didn't want to make him feel any more anxious than he already was. He didn't appear to be listening to me at all – wouldn't make much eye contact but mum reported later that he repeated more- or- less everything I had said to him on the car journey home!

Session2:

Michelle had told me that Ethan, although he hadn't *actually eaten* any new foods during that week following the first session, he appeared to be far less anxious around food (the result I wanted!) and I always tell mums that getting rid of the anxiety around eating is the first step.

Ethan was a lot more open with me – playing games with me and putting a glove puppet on and having a fight with the one I had on! (funny how kids love doing that with glove puppets isn't it!). He talked to me (via the glove puppets – *Marvin Monkey* and *Tommy Tiger*). A technique I use with children to get them communicating! He told me Marvin monkey was scared of trying new food.

I told him a little story about some magic flowers that had super powers that could help him not feel so scared around food. He took some of my special magic flowers home and of course they helped him not to be scared!

Session 3:

Michelle reported back to me that Ethan had started eating new foods! He was still *cautious* of certain foods but his general anxiety around eating had really subsided. We did a little more *day dreaming* on purpose using his imagination to think about how easy it is to eat new things).

He brought his reward chart in to show me and it was lovely to see his little face light up with pride when he explained how he had achieved all his gold stickers!

Session 4:

Ethan's mum had spoken to me during the week to say that Ethan was now "eating almost normally" but she was worried that after the sessions had finished he may just go back to his old ways.

This is what we all worry about as mums isn't it! However, I assured her that if she followed my three rules – to stay **Consistent**, **Persistent** and **Patient** – he would be fine!

I explained to Michelle that if *she* stayed *assertive* with Ethan, not giving him too big a choice for his lunch or tea, and stayed *consistent* in her efforts at mealtimes – he would continue to progress.

Ethan continued to try new foods every week – of course some he liked – some he didn't – that's normal! But.... in general, he moved forward with no fear of food whatsoever.

The little boy who sat in my office on that first therapy session and said nothing had turned into a happy little chappy who was prepared to try any food mum put in front of him.

Even though Ethan's eating hadn't been that severe when he first came to see me – it could have so easily turned into a case of a child with ARFID/SED. By easing the anxiety – we averted what could have very soon become - an eating disorder.

What Ethan's mum says:
Ethan was a totally normal eater until he choked on some dry baby snacks one day, it took so long to

dislodge the obstruction that he started to go blue. We managed to get it out finally. With the panic over for us, Ethan must have remembered this frightening experience because he then started to gag and choke on lots of things regularly after that. He was only just 2 years old and this was the start of his fear of food.

In time, the foods he would comfortably eat were limited to only the following:

Breakfast: Toast with vegemite

Lunch: vegemite sandwich

Dinner: Fish fingers, breaded chicken, chips occasionally, plain pasta occasionally, plain pizza

Other: Petit Filous, Ella's fruit pouches, crisps, plain biscuits, plain cakes, pieces of cheese.

He would eat nothing else and when something new was put in front of him he would melt down, when being encouraged to try other foods he would cry, shake, gag, choke, try to make himself vomit.

Clearly, Ethan loved Elaine from the start, He didn't want to leave, he ate her crisps, chatted with her, listened to her stories and even had a gift of a sticker chart.

Elaine encouraged me to share the Tiger came to tea story at home and act it out using one new food at a time in tiny quantities. We did this once a week for a few weeks. We included his older sisters as Elaine had suggested, we all had fun and very quickly, by our second Tea party session Ethan was nibbling at small pieces of apple.

Within 2 months the choking and gagging had stopped, he was slowly trying new things.

Still no veg and barely any fruit but all of these new foods he now loved: Rice, pasta with plain sauce, cheese sandwiches, sausages, bagels, pancakes.

By about 6 months after sessions Ethan was now loving meatballs, chicken breast, roast dinners, scampi, ham sandwiches, pieces of apple and raw carrot, sometimes a little cucumber and he loves cabbage.

Although Ethan is still funny about milk in cereal and bits in sauces, and hardly eats any fruit and veg, his food range is huge now and he is like almost any other regular 5-year-old boy. Elaine is constantly in touch with me, checking on Ethan's Progress, always making time to check he's still on track.

We are a family that loves to eat out, and with 2 teenage girls who eat everything, going out for meals was quite challenging with Ethan until he turned about 3, a year after therapy with Elaine. Now at 5 years old, we are out at least once a week enjoying family meals to Indian, Chinese, Mexican, any type of restaurant we fancy.

Our biggest challenge before was going to a carvery on a Sunday for a Roast, which is now one of Ethan's favourite things to do.

Ethan's comments
I felt shy at first....

Elaine made me feel like I was wondering what was going to happen but I was excited to find out.

I liked her room it was comfy, especially the big chair for me, I liked her stories, especially The Tiger came to Tea because mummy then bought the book and we could play tea parties at home.

Elaine gave me a sticker chart, which I like.

I want to go back and see Elaine again because I saw her not long ago when my sister Sophie went and she's really nice, but my mummy says now that I eat all the foods I don't need to see Elaine anymore, but I still want to.

What Are The Alternatives For SED Kids?

Elaine: Before we discuss the alternatives –
I want to make it clear that
Selective Eating Disorder or
ARFID (Avoidant, Restrictive
Food Intake Disorder) as it is
known in the USA is now included
in the DSM-V because the
American Psychiatric Association
have finally recognised it as a true
eating disorder.

The first thing a mum or dad will
do when they realise their child has
a problem with food and eating is
to take him to the GP.

Now, there could be a very valid reason why their child is refusing to eat certain foods – it may be that he has recently choked on something and it's caused him to be fearful of repeating that experience, or it could be that he, as a toddler, suffered with reflux and his subconscious remembers that and is almost trying to protect him by preventing him from eating.

Obviously depending on the age of the child he may or may not be able to tell you why he can't eat. The normal response from the child is that they are "scared" of eating but they can't usually tell you why. Mainly because in their conscious mind they *don't* know why.

It's the subconscious that holds the memories, the fears, the anxieties.

So…. mum takes the child to the GP. The GP says not to worry. She may go back two, three, four times before the doctor may refer the child to CAMHS (Child and Adolescent Mental Health Services)

The unfortunate thing is that there is usually a 9-12 month waiting list to see a CAMHS mental health Professional, so by the time the child does get seen – the situation is usually quite critical.

The child may or may not have lost a lot of weight (depending on the type of safe foods he is eating)

Naturally if he is eating a lot of white/beige foods, i.e. carbs, then he won't have lost weight. However, if his nutrition has been so low that he has lost a vast percentage of his body weight, he may be taken in to hospital and fed via a gastric tube.

One of the main reasons why treatment from the medical professionals, dieticians and nutritionists has *not* proved successful with children suffering with SED is that the child actually has a *phobia*....an aversion to eating. Just like someone has a phobia for spiders, or flying, or high buildings.

The child's fear of food is just as authentic as all other phobias.

Of course, the best way to treat a phobia is to change that mindset – to get to the subconscious mind and change those memories, those thoughts, and those feelings. This is why hypnosis plays a huge part in a child's recovery from SED.

What we have to be aware of is the fact that unless the child has reached a stage whereby he is at medical risk i.e. he has malnutrition and is losing a lot of weight, he is not actually "ill" – he has a phobia.

But what happens of course, once the child has been to see the GP and is now labelled with selective eating disorder, he is then treated as a sick child, probably both at home and at school.

The child undoubtedly gains a lot of attention from those around him – mum, dad, grandparents, teachers, dinner ladies, friends of the family etc… and now that child is getting so much attention – does he really want to lose it?

This of course is not the case for *all* children with SED but it's worth thinking about this when setting off on a course of treatment/ therapy.

If a child comes to me with SED or even simply picky eating, I treat them in exactly the same way. I treat the anxiety and use some subliminal hypnosis and talking therapy to change his thoughts about food.

Mistakes, Myths and Misunderstandings to Avoid

Jonathan: Okay. What, around getting your child to eat, do you think is the number one myth, that old wives' tale, that's false?

#1 Myth: No child will starve

Elaine: Yes. Okay. I think the biggest myth is that no child will starve. You'll get people saying, "Oh, don't worry about him. He won't starve. He'll eat. Send him to bed without his tea. If he's not going to eat it, send him to bed. He'll have his breakfast. He's not going to starve."

Well, that is the biggest myth, because of course children do starve. They get so phobic about food they will not eat at all. You can promise that child the earth. You could promise him to go to Disney World for a month. He would not eat. That's probably the biggest myth that I've come across, really.

In my opinion, the *biggest myth is that no child will starve*, because I get a lot of mums say to me that various people have said to them, "Oh, don't worry. *He won't starve*. He'll eat eventually."

Well, actually that isn't true. The phobic child will **not** eat. We're talking about a child with such a ***severe phobia*** of food that he's not going to eat. If he's dropped his safe foods down, and down, and down until he's not eating any solids, he will starve, and it will take medical intervention to get that child well again.

#1 Mistake: They're not naughty

Jonathan: What would you say is the biggest mistake that people make?

Elaine: I think the biggest mistake is that they think the child is naughty.

You know, other people think that the child's just being naughty. You could be out in a restaurant. It's happened to me, when my own daughter was being fussy in the restaurant. You hear people saying, "Oh, if it was my daughter, I'd force her to eat that." Or, "I'd give her a slapped bottom," or something. You know?

Because they think the child is being naughty because she's refusing to eat, and of course it's not.

The child has got a phobia, and it's a bit like if I said to you, "Here you are, darling. Here's a lovely plate of worms and cockroaches. Eat them up. They're delicious." What would you say? You'd say, "No. No, I'm not eating those. They're horrible. Disgusting." *That's what the child sees when he sees ordinary food.*

If we can put it in that context, then you get to the idea that the child isn't being naughty. He's just phobic. He's just emotionally anxious about food.

#1 Misunderstanding: Behavioural change is easy

Jonathan: Elaine, what do you think the biggest misunderstanding about helping children to eat is?

Elaine: I think the biggest misunderstanding is that they can change very quickly, their *behaviour* can change very quickly, because children are all unique, and what works for one child, doesn't necessarily work for another, or it might not work so quickly.

For example, I had a child recently who after just one session, just started eating lots of different foods. That was great, but it doesn't happen like that all the time.

It does take a little bit of work. It depends on the child's environment, depends on the family life, the dynamics in the family, how many people are on that team, as it were, helping the child to eat.

It could be that there is just a single mum and the child, and perhaps that single mum and the child just sit and have their dinner on their own every day.

The child doesn't see a lot of food on the table, because it's just his and mum's.

There's lots of different dynamics, and I think what we have to understand is that some children react quicker than others, and some ... Well, I wouldn't say that a child is slow. That doesn't sound right, but what I'm trying to say is that sometimes it's actually better that it goes a bit more slowly, and they do things in stages.

Going back to my **consistence**, **persistence**, and **patience**, that would come into it as well, because of course you do need to be *consistent* with a child. You do need to be *persistent*. You do have to have a little bit of authority with them to push them, to get them eating, and of course you have to be *patient*.

Massive Motivation

Jonathan: What are the major rewards we can
            expect from helping out our child,
            to get our child to eat?

Have Happier Mealtimes

Elaine: I think the major reward is that
            you're going to have a happier
            mealtime, to start with. I mean,
            that's the big thing, isn't it? Let's
            face it.

            Mealtimes should be happy. They
            should be relaxed. They should be
            calm. They should be nice. You
            should be able to sit and chat.

That's going to be one of the major rewards, and to be able to take their children out to eat as well, out to restaurants, and going on holiday, and all that travelling, and that's one of the major rewards I think.

Get Your Child Eating

Jonathan: What else?

Elaine: Really, with mum and dad working off the same page, the child is now eating normally. The child, the brothers and sisters are perhaps not ridiculing the little one anymore about his eating, and the selective eating disorder child isn't getting all that attention, because it affects the whole family, doesn't it?

You've got the other siblings who are not getting the attention that the selective eating disorder child is getting, so they're probably playing up as well in certain ways, you know? Being naughty, not going to bed properly. You can have a whole sort of general happy family, really, I think.

Jonathan: The whole family gets happier?

Elaine: Mm-hmm yes! The whole family will be happier.

Jonathan: Fabulous. What seems, with your clients and the feedback that you've had over the many years that you've been doing this now, what is the number one reward that people seem to get most excited about and the happiest about?

Enjoy a Fuller Future

Elaine: I think it's really just that they can see a future that's going to be happier, to be honest with you.

They can see themselves going on holiday and not having to worry about taking a suitcase full of baked beans or something.

They can see that they can go out to lunch with friends and not have, perhaps, one of the friends mentioning that the child's got a food problem, and causing a bit of tension at the table. Basically, every mealtime is not going to be a nightmare for them.

They can see that future as happy, and they can know that that child, the child that had the eating disorder, is going to grow into a wonderful little human being, emotionally and physically.

Jonathan: Well, Elaine, thanks very much for that. And I hope I'm not labouring the point but I'm sure there are mum's and dads, and of course anyone else who's reading this or listening to it or indeed watching it, will no doubt be very interested in finding out even more. So, let's tell people where to find you mostly...

http://GetYourChildEating.com
Elaine's Facebook group.
Get Your Child Eating tutorial training online, that people can register to find out about on the web site or of course, on the HypnoArtsApp where they can join our Life Changing Experiences Book Club.

Meet Elaine

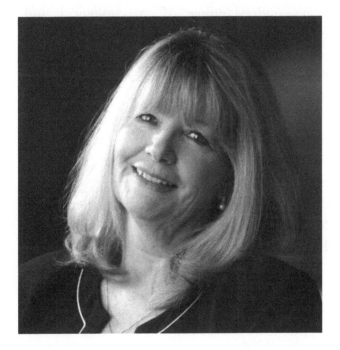

Elaine Hodgins is an expert in Childhood Psycho-Therapy, (CPT), whose accomplishments include training as a general registered nurse where she worked primarily in paediatrics for many years. Taught aviation medical training to pilots and cabin crew for a major airline, and has spent the past 15 years as a clinical Hypnotist and Psychotherapist, again working primarily with children and teens.

Elaine won the prestigious Pat Lucas TV award when she was a children's nurse for "The understanding of psychological and emotional needs of children in hospital" And recently in business won her BNI chapter "Oscar" for giving a star presentation on children's eating disorders.

She sees 25-30 children every week at her two clinics at Harley Street in London and Woodley in Berkshire, and all her work with children comes from referrals from other happy Mums, Dads and Carer's of kids with Picky Eating Problems.

Postword

Hi there, it's Jonathan Chase.

I'm incredibly lucky because as Director and Interviewer for HypnoArts Partnership Publishing, I'm allowed to be Midwife to some awesome people's ideas, expertise and treasures being shared with the world.

Elaine Hodgins is incredibly experienced with helping children overcome their eating disorders, as many happy parents will bear testament too.

Getting your child to eat gives the whole family more peace of mind, protecting the child's future health as well as the health of family relationships. Let Elaine help you get your child eating

Envoi: This is a 'Postword'.

Unlike a foreword I'm not here to tell you to read the book; I'm here to tell you to read it again, and again.

As with all #HypnoArtsBooks you should be able to do that on an average commute into town, definitely while you're waiting for your cancelled flight, or over a couple of lunches.

Our authors don't do fluff or fancy passages full of rhetoric, we don't do the 'bigger the book the better the content' thing.

So go back and read it again. Make notes in the margins. Fold page corners to mark the best bits. Spill coffee and tea on the cover...

READ the book and allow it to help your life change. Enhance Your Experience and boost your business now.

Acknowledgements

With Thanks

Cover Photography by *Saskia Bregazzi*
@shewhosewsuk

Author Photographs by *Gary Wheal -*
GoosebumpsPhotography.com

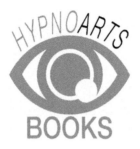

HypnoArts Publications

Enhancing the Experience of Life

For the most up to date information on;
Books, Audio, Courses and Video Tutorials,
Author information, links to forums
and FaceBook groups Live Author Appearances and events
download the free #HypnoArts App
from iTunes App Store or Google Play

or Visit **HypnoArts.com**
and grab your copy of our email newsletter.

We look forward to meeting you.
Jane Bregazzi. CEO HypnoArts

Lightning Source UK Ltd.
Milton Keynes UK
UKHW02f1837280518
323360UK00008B/319/P

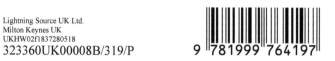